Banana Benefits: 20 Health And Wellness Benefits That Come From Eating A Banana A Day

Table of Contents

Introduction

There are different types of banana available in the world today. There are the raw bananas which are starch in nature and they are referred to as plantain and there is the banana fruit. The plantains are green in color while the banana fruit is yellow in color. Everyone has come across a banana the fruit. They are one of the most readily available fruits, yet they are the most ignored. Despite its many health benefits, banana fruit is one of the less consumed fruits in the world.

There are many reasons why some people dislike eating bananas. Some people hate the bananas because they think it is a baby food. Other dislike them because they have brown spots in them but despite the reason you might hate the bananas, the fruits is rich in nutrients that are of great benefit to your body. It is thus important for you to know the health benefits that are associated with the fruits.

Health Benefits Of Eating Bananas Everyday

Just like other fruits, bananas are rich in nutrients and they offer you great health benefits.

1. Rich In Potassium

Bananas are rich in potassium which is one of the important minerals required by the body. Potassium is one of the blood electrolytes together with sodium and the chloride. The electrolytes are responsible for carrying the electoral charge which helps to maintain and regulate the fluid balance in the body. Potassium also helps in regulating your heart beat. Potassium is an integral part of all the cells as it is required for the growth of the cells. It acts as a catalyst in many of the biological reactions especially during the release of the energy. Potassium is needed for the production of the insulin in the pancreas. This will help in regulating the blood sugar. Potassium together with sodium helps in regulating the blood pressure in the body.

2. Contains Vitamin B6

Vitamin B6 is one of the water soluble vitamins required in the body. This means that the vitamin is not stored by the body and you will have to take it on a daily basis. If you take excess of the vitamin your body will automatically flash the excess away. The Vitamin B6 is vital in your body it works as a co-enzyme in many of the biological functions. It is very important for the process of deamination (this is a process of removing an amine group from a molecule) and transamination.

The vitamin helps in maintaining a healthy brain function. This is because vitamin B6 helps make the neurotransmitters that carry signals from one cell to another. Vitamin B6 also helps in improving your mood by promoting the production of the serotonin and norepinephrine hormones that influence your mood. It also promotes the production of melatonin which helps to maintain and regulate the body clock. Vitamin B6 helps in the formation of red blood cells that are used for the transportation of oxygen across the body. It also helps in the breakdown of the proteins. Though there is no enough evidence, the vitamin has been reported to help in reducing the heart disease. It also helps in regulating the morning sickness (nausea and vomiting) in pregnant women.

3. Rich In Manganese

Manganese is a vital element in the body. It helps in the normal functioning of the skeletal and connective tissue. Manganese also acts as a catalyst and also forms essential enzymes that are involved in the synthesis of the amino acids and cholesterol. It helps in the metabolism of carbohydrates. Manganese helps in the formation of a healthy bone structure. It promotes the absorption of calcium in the body. It enables the proper functioning of the thyroid gland and the sex hormones. It also helps in regulating the blood sugar level.

4. Contains Vitamin C

Vitamin C is one of the most popular vitamins. It is one of the easily digested and absorbed vitamins. It is one of the water soluble vitamin and you are required to take the vitamin daily for the normal functioning of the body. Vitamin C is important in the formation of dentine (layer of the tooth). The vitamin is also important in the metabolism of tyrosine which is a non-essential amino acid. Tyrosine is a building block of some of the important neurotransmitters. Vitamin C helps in the formation of collagen in the connective tissues. The collagen is a component that is use to bind the cells together. The collagen also helps in wound healing. The vitamin helps in promoting the utilization of the iron, follacin and calcium.

Vitamin C stimulates the formation of the bile which is required for digestion. It also acts as an antioxidant that saves our body from free radicals. It promotes a healthy immunity and also helps in lowering the blood pressure. Vitamin C helps to lower the level of toxicity in the body. Vitamin C has been reported to act as an antihistamine that helps in controlling colds. It also protects the skin from the UV light.

5. Contains Biotin

Bananas are rich in biotin which is a vitamin that is found in small amounts in different foods. Biotin helps to reduce the thinning of the hair and also brittle nail. Biotin is also an essential vitamin as it helps in promoting metabolism in the body. The vitamin also plays a role in the production of the blood glucose through breakdown of carbohydrates in the body

6. A Rich Source Of Copper

Copper is an element that is required for the normal functioning of the body. Copper helps in the promotion of proper growth. It is also required in the absorption and utilization of the iron. It acts as a catalyst in some of the enzymatic reactions. Copper help is the normal functioning of the connective tissues. It promotes the formation of the red blood cells in the body and also in the proper functioning of the thyroid gland. It also helps in promoting the health of the eyes by protecting them from macular degeneration and also helps in maintaining a healthy hair.

7. Contains Fiber

As mentioned above, bananas are very rich in fiber which helps you to remain full for long. This will help you in reducing the amount of food you will be taking. The bananas also help you to control the sugar cravings. This is because once you eat a banana your body will not need the sugar. The fiber in the bananas will help in reducing constipation as the transit time will be reduced and the fecal output will be increased. The good bacteria growth is stimulated by the fiber. The bacteria help in inhibiting pathogens.

8. The Bananas Will Help In Reducing Colorectal Cancer

The colorectal cancer includes colon cancer, rectal cancer or the bowel cancer. This is done by the fiber contained in the bananas. The fiber promotes the production of the volatile fatty acids namely; butyric, acetic and lactic acid and reduces the pH and the concentration of the ammonia in the colon. This will reduce the fermentation of the carbohydrates

9. The Bananas Help In Reducing Risk Of Heart Disease

The vitamins and minerals mentioned above helps in reducing the risk of heart disease. The fiber contained in the banana also helps in reducing the heart disease by lowering the levels of the cholesterol in the body. It does this by promoting the production of the High Density Lipoproteins that usually take the excess cholesterol away from the heart and the body cells into the liver.

10.   It Reduces The Chances Of Breast Cancer

It has been reported that the bananas helps to reduce the risk of breast cancer. This is because of the fiber that reduces the bio-availability of the estrogen in the body by binding the circulating hormone.

11.   The Bananas Help To Alleviate Stomach Ulcers

Bananas have been reported to have an antacid effect; this usually helps to control the acid in the body which prevents heartburn. Since the acid will be under control, the stomach lining will be protected from erosion which will prevent the stomach ulcers. Another way that bananas help in preventing the stomach ulcers is by promoting the cells in the stomach lining to produce a thicker protective mucus that helps in protecting the stomach from the acid.

12.   The Banana Provides Energy

As seen above the fruit is rich in nutrients which once they are absorbed they will provide energy. Bananas are also rich in sugar that is converted to energy once it is digested.

13.   Good For The Skin

Eating the fruit is beneficial but also the banana peels are also very important. The peels have been reported to help in maintaining a good skin. The skins can treat skin conditions like acne and psoriasis.

14.   It Can Be A Hangover Cure

Taking a banana in the morning after a night of drinking will help you to reduce the hangover. The bananas usually replenish the electrolytes especially the potassium that were lost because of the alcohol.

15.   Improve The Electrolytes Loss

Diarrhea is one of the major causes of electrolytes elimination in the body. Once you start taking the bananas, your electrolytes levels will get back to normal. The bananas usually replenish the levels of potassium which will help to maintain the fluid balance. The bananas are rich sources of pectin which is a compound that helps in regulating the digestion reducing constipation. The fiber as mentioned above helps to promote the growth of the good bacteria in the body which will helps in fighting bacteria like E.Coli which causes diarrhea.

16.   Promotes Healthy Kidney

The maintaining of the fluid balance in the body through potassium will help to protect the kidneys. The bananas also help in reducing kidney cancer through the phenolic compounds as they contain high amounts of these compounds.

17.   Helps In Building Strong Bones

Bananas will help you promote the building of healthy and strong bones. This is because the nutrient contained in the bananas help in the absorption of calcium which is the building block of bones and teeth.

18.   The Bananas Helps You To Stop Smoking

Taking bananas on a daily basis will help you to reduce the nicotine addiction. The bananas are very beneficial especially to persons who are in the process of quitting the nicotine. This is because the potassium, manganese and Vitamin B6 will help you fight the effects of nicotine withdrawal.

19.   Bananas Helps In Fighting Addiction

In the brain there is a neurotransmitter that is responsible for the addiction. The neurotransmitter is called dopamine. Dopamine plays a role in the reward-motivated behavior that brings about addiction. The intake of bananas affects the production of dopamine in the brain especially to persons who have the amino acid tyrosine deficiency. This will help in reducing the addiction. The prevention of dopamine production might also negatively affect your mood as the neurotransmitter is also responsible for the mood and good feeling.

20.　　Bananas Helps To Increase The Sex Drive

Bananas are rich sources of vitamins that are responsible for the production of the sex hormones. Manganese promotes the production of the sex hormones which generally improves the sexual function.

Apart from the nutrients benefits, there are other ways that you may use the banana externally to promote wellness.

- You may use the banana to moisturize your skin. If you have a dry skin, you can mash the bananas in a bowl and apply them on your skin. Leave it for 20 minutes and rinse it off. For the oily skin, mix the mashed bananas with lemon and apply it on your body. The lemon will reduce future oil production through Vitamin C.

- The banana can be a good remedy for your itchy scalp; potassium in the banana promotes this effect. For successful results it is advisable for you to use the banana in combination with other foods like avocado and yogurt. Mix the three ingredients together and blend them.

Apply the mixture on your scalp and rinse after 20 minutes with warm water

- It can be used to fight wrinkles; use the mixture between avocado and banana as anti-aging cream. Avocados are rich in Vitamin E which is known for promoting smooth skin and preventing the formation of age spots.

- Helps to remove the dead skin; scrubbing your skin especially the facial skin will help to remove the dead cells and give you a smooth skin.

- Helps to soften cracked heels; the bananas can help you have a smooth heel if you use it regularly. Apply the bananas on your cracked heels daily.

- It has been reported that the bananas can help to reduce puffy eyes; this is thorough the potassium which helps in promoting fluid retention.

- Can treat acne; applying the banana peels on your affected area daily will help to reduce the pimples. The peels can also help in reducing the skin warts.

Tips Of Including Bananas In Your Daily Diet

Eating bananas on a daily basis offers great benefits for your body. There are many ways that you can choose to eat the banana. Below are some tips that can help you to eat banana on a daily basis.

- Choose a ripe banana; this is one of the reasons why some people don't like the bananas. The banana might be yellow but not sweet this is usually because the starch has not yet been converted to sugars. The best banana to choose is the dark yellow banana with no green patches (ensure that the banana is completely yellow from tip to the bottom).

- If you don't like the banana as a whole, you might choose to make a fruit juice. Take a few fruits and add the banana and mix them together

- Making a smoothie is one if the great ways of taking the banana fruit. There are many smoothie recipes that you may choose from.
- Bake cakes; you may choose to incorporate the banana as an ingredient when you are baking the cake.

- Making a fruit salad can also be a fun way of eating your banana; you can mix the banana with some of your favorite fruits.

Examples Of Recipes

There are many ways you can choose from when it comes to eating your bananas. Below are a number of recipes that you can use.

This is one of the creative ways of taking your banana. The cake is a three layer cake that can be enjoyed by 12 people.

Ingredients

- 2 cups of cream

- 2 ¼ cups white sugar

- ½ cup of water

- ¼ cup cubed butter

- 1 ¼ tea spoon of salt

- 2 ¼ cup unsalted butter

- 1 ½ cups of mashed bananas

- 3/4 cups of brown sugar

- 3 large eggs

- 3 tea spoon vanilla

- 1 ½ cups of milk

- 3 cups of all- purpose flour

- 1 ½ tea spoon baking soda

- 1 ½ of powdered sugar

Directions

- ### To Make The Caramel Sauce

Take the cream and warm it over low heat and don't let it boil. Take 1 ½ cups of the white sugar and mix it with water. Stir it until all the sugar dissolves. Bring the mixture to a boil stirring it until it obtains a deep brown color. Pour the cream in the mixture immediately. Add the cube butter and the ½ a tea spoon of the salt and whisk the mixture until it is smooth. Return the mixture to the fire and heat in low heat for 5 minutes. Pour the mixture into a jar and refrigerate.

- ### To Make The Caramel Butter Cream

Take ½ cup of the already made caramel sauce, ½ cup of the unsalted butter, 1 tea spoon of vanilla and ¼ tea spoon of salt and put them in a bowl. Mix the ingredients using a hand mixer until they are smooth and fluffy. Add the powdered sugar slowly and mix them until smooth.

- ### To Make The Banana Cake

Pre heat the oven to 325°F. Then take a mixer (A bowel and hand mixture will do) put in the remaining unsalted butter, brown sugar and the remaining white sugar (3/4 cups) mix them until they are fluffy. Add the eggs one by one and beat them until they are silky. In a separate bowel pour in the flour, baking soda, salt and whisk them. Then add the vanilla, mashed bananas whisk them and pour the mixture to the egg mixture. Take three cake pans, grease them and pour the cake mixture into the pans in equal amount. Pour the caramel sauce into each of the three pans, swirl them with a knife and bake for 40 minutes. Cool the pans on a rack before removing the cakes.

When all the cakes have cooled down, take the cake and place the bottom layer on a plate. Spread the cake with a butter cream. Repeat this for all the three cakes. Once the whole cake is assembled, pour the remaining caramel sauce on top of the cake and garnish the cake with banana slices. Enjoy with a cold drink.

If you enjoy taking bread in the morning, then this might be the right choice for you.

Ingredients

- 6 medium over ripe bananas (mashed)

- 2 cups of all-purpose flour

- 1 tea spoon of baking soda

- ¼ tea spoon of salt

- ½ cup butter

- 1 tea spoon cinnamon

- 2 eggs (beaten)

- ¾ cup of brown sugar

Directions

Pre heat the oven to 350°F and grease a loaf pan. Take a large bowl and pour in cinnamon, flour, baking soda and salt. Mix the ingredients together. In a separate bowl, mix butter and sugar until smooth. Stir the bananas and the eggs until, they are blended together then pour the mixture into the flour mixture. Pour the batter into the loaf pans. Bake for 60- 65 minutes until the knife inserted into the center comes out clean. Let the bread cool before removing it.

This can be enjoyed as a snack.

Ingredients

- 2 ripe bananas

- 12 ice cubes

- 2 table spoon of vanilla kefir (drinkable yogurt)

- ½ tea spoon of cinnamon

- 1/8 tea spoon of ground nutmeg

- 1/8 tea spoon of ground allspice

Directions

Take the vanilla kefir, bananas (chopped) and all the other ingredients and put them in a blender. Blend until the mixture is smooth. Serve immediately.

Ingredients

- 1 cup of sugar

- ¼ cup of corn starch

- 2 eggs beaten

- ½ tea spoon of salt

- 3 tea spoons of butter

- 1 ½ tea spoons of vanilla extract

- 2 large ripe bananas

- 1 pastry shell baked

- 1 cup of heavy whipping cream

Directions

In a large bowel, put in sugar, corn starch, salt, milk mix them until they are smooth. Put the mixture in to a sauce pan and stir over a medium heat until the mixture is thickened and bubbly. Remove from the heat and pour in the eggs, return to the heat for about 2 minutes stirring gently. Remove from the heat and pour in the vanilla and the butter and stir. Cover the mixture with a plastic wrap and refrigerate for 30 minutes. Take the pastry shell and spread them across the mixture and slice the bananas and arrange them over the filling. Spread the whipped cream and refrigerate for 6 hours.

Ingredients

- 1 ½ cups of vanilla ice cream

- ¾ cups of milk

- 2 table spoons of unsweetened cocoa

- 2 bananas sliced

- ½ table spoon of vanilla

- Whipped cream (optional)

- Candy bar (choose your favorite)

Directions

In the blender; pour in the ice cream, milk, cocoa, banana and vanilla. Blend the ingredients until they are smooth. Pour the shake into the glass and top with the whipped cream and the chosen candy bar

For the ice cream lovers this can be a good choice. All you need are two ingredients

Ingredients

- 1 ripe banana peeled and chopped

- 1 table spoon of sliced almonds

Directions

Freeze the banana and puree in a food processor. Pour the ice cream in the cup and top with almonds

Ingredients

- 2 ½ cups of all-purpose flour
- 2 tea spoons of baking powder
- ½ tea spoon of salt
- 1 cup white sugar
- 2/3 cups of butter (softened)
- 2 eggs
- 1 tea spoon vanilla extract
- 1 cup of mashed bananas
- 2 cups of semisweet chocolate cookies

Directions

Pre heat the oven 400°F and grease the cookie sheets. Take a mixing bowl and sift the flour, baking powder and salt together. On a separate bowel cream the butter with sugar until light and fluffy. Beat the eggs and mix with vanilla pour in the mashed bananas and mix together. Pour the mixture in to the flour mixture and stir until they are combined. Pour in the chocolate chip cookies. Put the mixture in to the already prepared cookie sheets and bake them for 15 minutes. Remove them and let them cool. Enjoy with a glass of milk or juice.

www.ingramcontent.com/pod-product-compliance
Lightning Source LLC
Chambersburg PA
CBHW061948280526
45787CB00004B/1777